Medical Cannabis
Initial Medical Consultation

A Guide for Patients

by

J. Kimber Rotchford, M.D., M.P.H.

This book expresses the views of J. Kimber Rotchford, M.D., a specialist in treating patients suffering from chronic pain and substance use disorders. As well he is a Fellow of the American College of Preventive Medicine.

The book is published by Olympas Medical Services, Ltd. of Port Townsend, Washington. Printed in The United States of America.

First Edition May 2018

Cover Art is reproduced from private collection of author.
Front Cover by Elisabeth Haight (www.elisabethhaight.com)
Back Cover *James K Dragon* by Maggie Roe

ISBN-13: 978-1717018120
ISBN-10: 1717018122

Contact the Publisher:
Olympas Medical Services, Ltd.
1136 Water St. Suite 107
Port Townsend, WA 98368
www.OPAS.us
staff@OPAS.us

This book can be ordered from Amazon and purchased at retail stores

Purchasers of this book are invited to download a PDF copy with clickable links at DrRotchford.com/guide

Medical Cannabis
Initial Medical Consultation

A Guide for Patients

by

J. Kimber Rotchford, M.D., M.P.H.

TABLE OF CONTENTS

Introduction

This "initial consultation" is for those who are considering using cannabis for medical purposes. It addresses the important elements a capable physician will likely review during an initial consultation to evaluate and authorize the use of medical cannabis. American physicians are still not legally able to prescribe cannabis. Except for marijuana, there is no other substance a physician can legally authorize, but not prescribe.

From the outset, patients who are authorized cannabis are acting on their own behalf when prescribing themselves cannabis products. Based on current federal laws, a patient writes their own prescription. A provider only authorizes its use. Because of the complexities of the human body, mind and spirit, it is advised to be prepared to carefully evaluate the pros and cons of using medicinal cannabis.

Historically, physicians have been considered uniquely qualified to inform patients of the indications, risks, and side effects from using any substance for medical purposes. Because of its longstanding status as an illegal drug, widespread ignorance regarding medicinal cannabis still persists. Synthetic dronabinol is an FDA-approved medication, and it mimics one of the more potent and active substances in cannabis products. Few physicians prescribe dronabinol (Marinol), in part because its FDA indications are limited to certain wasting conditions associated with cancer and AIDS. Furthermore, it is quite expensive and often not covered by third parties.

The treatment of conditions that respond to cannabis often benefit from additional therapeutic components. Perhaps the greatest risk from using medicinal cannabis is overlooking better therapeutic options? This is likely because cannabis is often effective in managing a broad range of symptoms. Other than when the over-use of cannabis has resulted in accidents, the most serious "side effects"commonly encountered in patients authorized to use cannabis are related to patients not using other effective and possibly safer care. In some cases, some of the overlooked modalities could substantially improve short as well as long-term health.

To avoid missing potentially essential medical care and to better assess the risks and benefits of medicinal cannabis, working with a qualified medical professional offers distinct advantages. A qualified medical professional can screen for hepatitis C and other conditions that complicate or render unsafe the use of cannabis products. In addition, professional support may be invaluable in addressing specific and associated general medical issues.

There is a common association between medical cannabis use and patients having elements of Post Traumatic Stress Disorder (PTSD). Hence, an entire chapter reviews the basics of understanding and care for PTSD. This publication can also help determine if regular cannabis use has become a substance use disorder (SUD), that is, the user has become addicted to cannabis products. An effective behavioral guide to recovering from a cannabis SUD as well as other substance use disorders is a chapter of its own and reflects a valuable resource by itself. Additionally, because oral use of cannabis is almost always recommended for medical purposes, options for home preparation of oral cannabis products is provided.

Note: most of the following discussions relate to what is considered the most active compound in cannabis products—Tetrahydrocannabinol, most commonly referred to as THC. A myriad of substances are found in natural cannabis products. Research into the plant's varied components, such as Cannabidiol (CBD), along with their unique risks and benefits, is rapidly progressing. The following discussion relates to natural cannabis products which have at least some THC in them.

Medical Cannabis by J. Kimber Rotchford, M.D.

CHAPTER ONE

Initial Medical Cannabis Consultation —A Guide for Patients

Welcome to the *Initial Medical Cannabis Consultation*. Whether you are considering the use of medical cannabis or wish to evaluate your existing cannabis experience, a consultation with a physician can be helpful to best determine whether medical cannabis can be a potentially safe and effective option. Unfortunately, finding physicians qualified to review the use of medical cannabis can be problematic.

Evaluating Risks Versus Benefits of Medical Cannabis

Evaluating the risks versus benefits of medical cannabis is the foremost consideration of the initial consultation. As with any medical prescription or use of a substance for medical purposes, the risks and benefits for cannabis are best determined by *each patient's* history and exam. This allows a practitioner to confirm or establish appropriate diagnoses and prognoses. The medical assessment is to be complemented by medical and pharmacological understandings. Professional oversight can establish effective dosing as well as discover any particular risks for side effects a patient could have.

Not everyone will benefit from cannabis nor will everyone suffer negative consequences. Thoughtful and safe use of cannabis requires, similar to other medical interventions, an appreciation of the possible benefits as well as the potential risks. Unfortunately, the historically recognized benefits and risks concerning medical cannabis are often **not** well supported by solid evidence. Rather, long-standing beliefs and prejudices often dominate assessments, even by professionals. Evidence-based research on medical cannabis has been compromised not only by legal impediments and social stigma, but also by the lack of financial incentives to do the research. Patents and other incentives to market standard pharmaceutical products based on FDA approval do not commonly exist with "natural" products such as cannabis products.

Benefits

While individualized care is best, medical cannabis does provide a therapeutic option for a number of medical conditions. Opinions diverge regarding which conditions are suitable for cannabis use. Randomized control trials are lacking, particularly those evaluating subsets of the population with a specific condition. Lack of robust evidence does not mean, however, that cannabis is not effective for a given condition. It simply means the evidence is lacking.

The following list of Washington State approved indications for authorizing medical cannabis is a good place to start in considering whether you have a condition likely to benefit from medical cannabis. Most of the items on the list have research or evidence which support the benefit of cannabis use. Other states have lists of approved indications including insomnia, depression, anxiety, panic attacks, harm reduction, slowing down dementia, muscle spasms, and more.

As already noted, cannabis products are particularly helpful in patients who have experienced significant traumas in their lives. These traumas may have been accidents, surgeries, serious illnesses, abuse, neglect and so on. Frequently, the associated and often subconscious memories related to trauma continue to interfere with health.

The parts of the human brain that remember and react to old traumatic memories are especially full of receptors that respond both to internally produced (naturally created by the brain)or externally consumed cannabinoids (derived from marijuana). Based on human neurophysiology, it is understandable that in patients who have been traumatized, THC would reduce anxiety, help with sleep, and promote better pain management. Patients with PTSD symptoms will often get dramatic relief from the use of THC containing products.. Nonetheless, they also will likely benefit from additional care. Given the prevalence of PTSD in patients who benefit from medical cannabis for chronic conditions, a more comprehensive discussion of PTSD follows in Chapter 3.

Recently, evidence indicates that cannabis can help limit the withdrawal from opioids and help control the dependence on opioids for pain management. With the recognized serious complications associated with opioid use and abuse, this indication alone is noteworthy.

In 2018, a physician licensed in the State of Washington may authorize medical cannabis for the following indications.

- Cancer

- Human immunodeficiency virus (HIV)

- Multiple sclerosis

- Epilepsy or other seizure disorder

- Spasticity disorders

- Intractable pain which is unrelieved by standard medical treatments and medications

- Glaucoma, either acute or chronic, limited for the purposes of this law to mean increased intraocular pressure unrelieved by standard treatments or medications

- Crohn's disease with debilitating symptoms unrelieved by standard treatments and medications

- Hepatitis C with debilitating nausea or intractable pain unrelieved by standard treatments or medications

- Chronic renal failure

- Post-traumatic stress disorder (PTSD)

- Traumatic brain injury

- Any disease, including anorexia, which results in nausea, vomiting, wasting, appetite loss, cramping, seizures, muscle spasms, and/or spasticity, when these symptoms are unrelieved by standard treatments or medications.

Risks (Side Effects) from Cannabis Use

Note: the following order of risks is not based on the severity of risk.

Addiction (Substance Use Disorder)

Cannabis use disorders (addiction) occur in about 10-15% of routine cannabis users and seem more common clinically the younger someone begins using cannabis. Cannabis use disorders are also more common in those who have smoked marijuana for years or suffer from other substance use disorders, whether the disorders are in remission or not. These other abused substances frequently include legal substance use disorders such as tobacco and alcohol use disorders. The brain's evolution and function often do not conform to current laws and regulations.

—The criteria for a substance use disorder (addiction) *(footnote)* include having at some of the following.

1. Tolerance/withdrawal
2. Cravings/preoccupation
3. Continued use despite harm
4. Loss of control and cognitive distortions or denial about associated problems.

Footnote: American Society of Addiction Medicine (ASAM) has helpful short and long definitions for addiction on their website under the resources tab:
https://www.asam.org/resources/definition-of-addiction

—The following questions may help you in determining whether you might be "addicted" to marijuana.

1. Have people close to you complained about your cannabis use?
2. Do you have problems with short-term memory?
3. Have you experienced paranoid episodes during cannabis use?
4. Do you find it difficult to get through a day without a joint?
5. Do you lack the energy to get things done the way you used to?
6. Do you ever worry about the effects of your cannabis use?
7. Do you have more difficulty in understanding new information?
8. Have you ever unsuccessfully attempted to cut down or quit?
9. Do you like getting stoned in the morning?
10. Are you spending more and more time stoned?
11. Do you experience craving, headaches, irritability, or difficulty concentrating when you cut down or cease cannabis use?
12. Do you continue to use cannabinoids despite memory deficits, lack of motivation, difficulty in recognizing and learning new patterns, relations with employers/supervisors, ability to think clearly, lower confidence levels, and less excitement/enthusiasm for life.

Although cannabis abuse is prevalent, animal studies show that cannabinoids do not seem to be as potent as other agents such as heroin, cocaine, and nicotine when it comes to causing a substance use disorder (addiction). One reason for this is that cannabinoids act as moderators of neuronal activity rather than direct neurotransmitters. In addition, they release less intense amounts of dopamine in the nucleus accumbens.

Further Notes on Addictions

As already noted, tobacco and alcohol use disorders are the SUDs most commonly associated with cannabis use disorders. Other patients sometimes have stimulant or opioid use disorders. It behooves cannabis users to be familiar with helpful ways to prevent and manage substance use disorders. Often poorly appreciated—even by some professionals—all SUDs share common findings, while also maintaining unique attributes. The treatment of SUDs is always best when individualized. See Chapter 6 for further behavioral ways to help with substance use disorders.

The average person associates addiction with physical dependence (for example, "that person is addicted to nasal decongestants"). The disease of addiction is something more than physical dependence. (*See footnote below*). The pathophysiology of addiction is associated with a release of dopamine in the reward centers of the brain. If a substance forces a release of dopamine in the reward system, it potentially can induce a substance use disorder.

Marijuana use, particularly when smoking it, is associated with a release of dopamine in the brain's reward system. The release is present, albeit less, when one uses comparable doses orally. Hence, cannabinoids, in particular THC, are potentially addictive substances. This has been

---

(Footnote): On Practical Pain Management's website there is an article written by the author, which further explores common confusion between physical dependence and addiction: Opioids: Addiction or Physical Dependence?
https://www.practicalpainmanagement.com/patient/resources/opioids-addiction-physical-dependence

demonstrated in laboratory studies as well as clinically. As already noted, current estimates are that 10-15% of regular users have a cannabis use disorder. A few people will actually become physically dependent on marijuana. They suffer withdrawal symptoms when its use is curtailed. Recently, the withdrawal from cannabis has been compared to a mild form of withdrawal similar to that experienced with opioids.

Surprisingly, clinical experience has revealed that overall recovery from other substance abuse disorders is **not necessarily** compromised by ongoing cannabis use and, in some instances, its use seems to help recovery from the abuse of alcohol and other substances. This comes as a surprise because historically it has been believed that outcomes with SUDs are best when all addictive substances are avoided. It is worth repeating that the best results for substance use disorders arise from individualized care—with the support of appropriately trained and experienced professionals.

Other Known Risks

—Cannabis is particularly risky in the context of active hepatitis C. We recommend anyone who uses cannabinoids regularly to be screened for hepatitis C, particularly those who are at higher risk. The baby boomer generation (born between approximately 1950 to 1965) are at higher risk as are those with a history of IV illicit drug use. It remains ironical that hepatitis C has been an indication for Medical Cannabis authorizations in Washington State. It's use is relatively contraindicated in the context of active or untreated hepatitis C.

—**Smoking marijuana** can lead to acute and chronic bronchitis, immunological impairment, and precancerous changes in the lungs.

—**Thought and Behavioral (Psychoactive) Side Effects can occur.** When one initially takes a standardized dose of orally consumed marijuana or whenever significant changes in serum levels arise, a cannabis effect is likely to be "felt." If one feels high, is paranoid, has the "munchies" (increased appetite), or is behaving differently, it is wise to avoid operating hazardous machinery, including automobiles. When marijuana is smoked, these activities are especially best avoided because rapid changes in blood levels of THC associated with smoking marijuana have been demonstrated to have significant cognitive and behavioral consequences. Both judgment and motor abilities can be compromised by cannabinoids, and measurable effects can linger for days after use.

When therapeutic serum levels of THC are stable, it becomes challenging to objectively measure cognitive or behavioral side-effects. Stable levels of THC also are likely to mitigate the addictive potential for using marijuana. This forms the basis of the strong recommendation I make for oral use only. See Dosing Instructions below.

More Discussion on Benefits and Risks

Addiction and abuse of cannabis gets widespread attention in our culture. Similarly, the use of cannabis in developing brains, up to the age of 25 in males, has demonstrated liabilities regarding brain development. For many reasons, regular use of cannabis is relatively contraindicated in youth and young adults.

In clinical practice, as experience shows, most patients seek help with cannabis for chronic painful conditions or appetite problems. Some seek help for sleep, anxiety, and symptoms related to PTSD. If they have never had a substance use disorder, whether with licit substances such as alcohol and tobacco or illicit substances, it is quite unlikely they will develop an addiction to cannabis. This is particularly true in patients who maintain stable levels through oral use only.

Cannabis products can provide potent symptomatic treatment. Nonetheless, it is always best to promote long-term healing or at least directly address the issues which cause the symptoms. Behavioral changes are frequently necessary, but formal medical or even surgical interventions can be indicated. When people start to feel safe, long-term changes and healing are more readily attained. Helping patients feel safer is perhaps the strongest benefit stemming from cannabis use.

Based on extensive clinical experience, a common risk or side effect of cannabis is related to patients getting distracted or not recognizing novel changes in their environment. This is particularly the case the day or so after using cannabis. Most people assume the risks are related to the levels of THC rising or reaching their peak serum levels. In my experience, significant risks also occur when the THC levels are going down. At this time, patients are perhaps even more prone to accidents, whether while driving or doing other activities. Consequently, serum levels of cannabis are best maintained either through routine oral or topical use. The exception would be for those concerns which are quite intermittent such as nausea and vomiting associated with chemotherapy.

In these cases, the peak effects associated with smoking marijuana makes sense.

While already reviewed to some degree, the following effects of cannabis warrant further discussion and references are available.

Cannabis Physical Dependence and Withdrawal

Abrupt cannabis termination in habitual users results in withdrawal symptoms similar to those from discontinuing opioids. The severity of withdrawal symptoms is dependent on the dose of THC consumed over time. Withdrawal is less likely to occur or symptoms are less when lower doses are consumed.

Haney M, Hart CL, Vosburg SK, Nasser J, Bennett A, Zubaran C, Foltin RW Neuropsychopharmacology. 2004 Jan; 29(1):158-70.

Cannabinoids and Sleep

The prevalence of sleep disturbance is high in patients with chronic pain and improved sleep equates well with improved pain management.

Opioids disrupt sleep[1] through a variety of mechanisms, but clearly aggravate or cause sleep apnea. While THC is a sedative, CBD is stimulating.[2] Higher doses of CBD can have sedating effects. THC alone had no effect on sleep quality, while adding CBD reduces stage 3 sleep and increases wakefulness.

---

[1] *Dimsdale JE, et al. J Clin Sleep Med, 2007, 3:33-36*

[2] *Dimsdale JE, et al. J Clin Sleep Med, 2007, 3:33-36*
    ***Nicholson A, et al. J Clin Pharmacol, 2004, 3:305-313*

Cannabis and Driving

States with medical marijuana laws have fewer traffic fatalities.[3]

—Fatality Analysis Reporting System 1985-2014

- Age 15-24 – 11% reduction

- Age 25-44 – 12% reduction

- Age 45 and older – no significant change

—Specific immediate reductions in States

- California – 16%

- New Mexico – 17.5%

There has been a gradual increase in motor vehicle accidents since marijuana legalization laws were passed. Mixing alcohol and cannabis creates significant impairment. As already discussed under dosing is an issue, while stable levels of cannabinoids are less likely to cause any impairment.

A person's judgment and motor abilities can be compromised by cannabinoids; moreover, the effects of cannabinoids can linger for at least days after use. If one is taking a standardized dose of **orally consumed** marijuana and changes in dosing levels occur or if one can feel medicated or directly feel a psychoactive effect, it is advisable to avoid operating hazardous machinery, including automobiles. If one has smoked marijuana, these activities are especially best avoided, unless the levels are stable.

---

[3] (Am J Pub Health, 2016 doi:10.2015/AJPH.2016.303577)

Patients who have been on a stable dose of orally consumed medical cannabis are likely safer drivers than if they were not on a stable dose of cannabis. When levels are stable over extended periods, it becomes difficult to measure cognitive impairment related to use. Cannabis when used with other substances such as alcohol or other psychoactive substances, whether prescribed or not, can have dramatic synergistic effects, for better and for worse! We generally screen for alcohol use and abuse and strongly advise patients who use cannabis to not mix it with alcohol or other substances when using machinery or driving.

Dosing and Route of Administration of Cannabis Products

As with all proper prescribing and use of a substance for medical purposes, whether natural or pharmaceutical, appropriate dosing is essential. Issues around dosing with natural products can be problematic due to the variety of substances involved and because concentrations can vary widely. Another complicating factor is the potential therapeutic synergy between the different cannabinoids found in the marijuana leaf or bud.

Some physicians prefer to prescribe dronabinol (Marinol) rather than authorized cannabis use. Dronabinol is basically pharmaceutical quality tetrahydrocannabinol (THC). Some third parties pay for it. The main advantage of pharmaceutical dronabinol is it allows for a confident and a relatively precise oral dose of THC. Nonetheless, even with "pharmaceutical grade" THC, absorption can vary significantly and patients' specific responses to doses vary significantly.

Some trial and error with dosing is commonly expected. Studies in rats have confirmed how important dosing is. Rats are readily averse to high doses and clearly prefer lower doses. Human cannabis smokers also report opposing effects.[4]

As with other substances, the route of administration also has direct effects on blood levels along with predictable therapeutic and toxic effects. Some physicians advise patients to use vaporizers to deliver cannabis products. The ease of use with vaporizers may facilitate appropriate dosing. When cannabis products are inhaled, the effects are more immediate and more readily adjusted. Vaporizing helps eliminate some of the irritative aspects of smoke and it may increase the assimilation of the various substances found in the marijuana plant. While these advantages are apparent, vaporizing is associated with higher levels of mind altering cannabinoids, which can fluctuate rather dramatically. These rapid changes and instability in serum levels, as previously noted, compromise brain function.

The intent of medical cannabis is to promote better functioning and well-being as with any medically prescribed substance. The brain likes homeostasis. That is, it prefers its internal environment to be stable. Based on pharmacology, when one smokes or vapes cannabis, unless

---

[4] *Braida D, Pozzi M, Cavallini R, Sala M*
Neuroscience. 2001; 104(4):923-6; Cheer JF, Kendall DA, Marsden CA
Psychopharmacology (Berl). 2000 Jul; 151(1)25-30.; Reilly D, Didcott P, Swift W, Hall
W Addiction.1998 Jun; 93(6):837-46.

doing so repeatedly throughout the day, it becomes challenging to maintain steady blood levels. In contrast, when taking it by mouth twice a day, or preferably three times a day, more stable levels can be achieved.

Granted, it is challenging to find the best oral dose. It can be 1-4 hours until one recognizes the peak effects of swallowed cannabis. Absorption can also be influenced by the amount of "fats" present in food consumed and other unrecognized variables. The bioavailability of cannabinoids range from 5-20 percent. A large 1st pass effect (breakdown) occurs from the liver, and erratic absorption from stomach and intestines exists. Nonetheless, if one carefully establishes a relatively steady concentration of cannabinoids whether in a food or tincture, one can most often readily find an effective dose without any side effects.

Sublingual delivery is an attractive alternative route of administration. A sublingual spray containing the cannabis-based extract (CBME) in combination with THC and CBD is currently approved in Canada for multiple sclerosis. The plasma levels achieved are similar to those of oral delivery but are more titratable and predictable (peak in about 1 hour; duration up to 4 hours).

One can also juice the leaves from fresh plants. By not heating or cooking the cannabis one can consume large amounts of therapeutic cannabinoids and be spared the concerns of psychoactive side effects.

By using food-quality glycerine, the patient (or cannabis tincture manufacturer) can readily extract active ingredients from the marijuana plant. Once extracted, the tincture has a relatively fixed concentration of active ingredients. Directions for creating your own tincture follow below in Chapter 4. The tincture can then be consumed as a set amount of drops, administered two or three times a day. By avoiding the need to heat the active ingredients, as with smoking, less intoxicating compounds (such as carboxylated THC) are formed and consumed. Oral use also avoids the side effects and concerns associated with smoking.

Patients commonly ask what percentage of different cannabinoids is best or what strains are best to use. Unfortunately, even within the same "strain" the diversity of compounds and strengths varies significantly. In addition, each brain has relatively unique receptors, and each condition treated is expected to have certain cannabinoids which are more likely to be safe and effective. Based on current research and inconsistencies in products, it is challenging to predict which strain or dose will work best in a given patient. Trial and error often remains the best option.

Many patients want to avoid THC entirely. As previously noted, however, THC has widespread therapeutic effects and may work synergistically with other cannabinoids and substances in marijuana. Indeed, for PTSD, pain management and other indications THC plays a valuable role. That being said, as already noted, the dose of THC should avoid feelings of having been medicated. . Another option, as already noted, is to utilize THC that has not been carboxylated through heating, as it then remains free of any significant psychoactive side effects. This is why drinking an entire glass of freshly squeezed leaves will not result in feeling "high." Currently and unfortunately, the juicing option remains expensive. The shelf life of fresh marijuana is quite short and a lot must be used to adequately get a full glass of juice

In summary, eventually studies may determine the safest and most effective doses and ways to use cannabis products. Until then, I routinely advise dosing by the oral route or to use topically applied cannabis. This way, cannabinoid levels are maintained relatively stable in the blood and it is challenging, perhaps impossible to measure cognitive deficits(brains not working well). When cannabis is used chronically and for medical purposes, the intent must be to improve brain function, not impair it!

CHAPTER TWO

Medical Cannabis—*A Physician's Experience*

Introduction

Cannabis has been legally authorized for debilitating and terminal conditions in the State of Washington since 1998. I have authorized medical cannabis to more than 1,000 patients. What follows are the findings based on this extensive clinical experience. Some of the particulars repeats the information and suggestions already provided in Chapter 1. However, some new data and comments have been included to support the benefits versus the risks of cannabis use in patients authorized to use under Washington State laws.

Patient Demographics

The average age of patients who seek a medical cannabis authorization is estimated to be in their early sixties. The youngest patient authorized was eighteen and the oldest was in their mid-90's. About two-thirds of the cannabis patients are male. Compared to patients in a general medical practice, these patients are more likely to live alone. Their income is likely below the median. Many are significantly disabled by intractable pain or the other qualifying conditions listed above. Nonetheless, about fifty percent are employed and some are quite successful in their work. Educational levels and race appeared consistent with other patients in the community.

Diagnoses

About ninety percent of the patients were authorized based on a diagnosis of intractable pain. The chronic pain conditions that benefit from cannabis are similar to those found in typical pain management practices: back pain, headaches, arthritis, neck pain, and fibromyalgia. The remaining 10 percent of patients were distributed among the other state-allowed, medical criteria. The majority had experienced limited therapeutic responses with conventional care or they had significant concerns about side effects. Indeed, recent evidence confirms that cannabis can limit the dependence on opioids for pain management.

Mental Health Diagnoses and Substance Use Disorders

An estimated fifteen percent of the patients would meet the criteria for a cannabinoid substance use disorder (SUD). Less than five percent, however, seemed to be seriously dependent. Comorbid SUDs are perhaps 25-50% more common in patients who routinely use cannabis products. Comorbid psychiatric conditions are common in complex chronic pain patients. As a result they are also relatively common in patients authorized to use cannabis for intractable pain.

Since cannabinoid receptors are implicated in remembering and responding to past trauma, the majority of patients who benefit significantly from cannabis use likely suffer from some degree of PTSD.

When a patient's sleep or pain is dramatically relieved by the occasional use of cannabis, it was predictive that the patient had experienced a significant traumatic event. As stated previously, a patient with a PTSD diagnosis may be greatly helped by medical cannabis. Nonetheless, they should examine all the available avenues for medical and behavioral treatment.

Follow-Up and Findings

As required by the law, patients must return to their authorizing physician for an annual review and a reauthorization. Of the returning patients, whom I've seen in practice (approximately 80%), an estimated five percent reported—or were found to have—difficulties attributable to cannabinoid use.

The most serious of these were lingering effects from hepatitis C complications. Cannabis use is known to aggravate the progression toward cirrhosis in patients with hepatitis C, reportedly more so than alcohol use. Nonetheless, hepatitis C has historically been an indication for cannabis use in Washington State. This is likely because of cannabinoids helping symptoms commonly associated with chronic hepatitis C.

A few patients had received driving under the influence charges (DUI's) related to THC found in their blood. Nonetheless, no apparent driving impairment specific to cannabis use was established. Based on pharmacology and brain physiology, significant impairment is **not** probable when blood levels of THC have been stable.

Results

About two-thirds of the cannabis patients demonstrated improvement in clinical markers associated with function, pain relief, or other symptoms. The progress can be dramatic in some cases. Most patients come to openly acknowledge that using cannabis by mouth, rather than smoking, works best. Patients understandably and frequently prefer to not "feel" anything. Some patients have stopped using cannabis, either because of side-effects, finances, resolution of symptoms, legal concerns, or other reasons.. These patients are roughly estimated to be about 20% of patients initially authorized.

Discussion

The clinical setting is often important when predicting outcomes. Many confounding variables could readily explain the above reported observations. Care which reflects compassion and is non-judgmental is likely to be an important variable. Through a respectful and therapeutic relationship, maintained over time, patients are better prepared to properly evaluate their relationship with, and the value of, their cannabis use. This is the same as for any chronically prescribed supplement, herbal remedy, or medication.

In conclusion, authorizing cannabis for medical reasons has been favorable. We can hope these observations lead to further research and dialogue on the merits of medical cannabis

CHAPTER THREE

Post-Traumatic Stress Disorder (PTSD)

As mentioned previously, medical cannabis is indicated in the treatment of PTSD. Because of the prevalence of PTSD in those seeking authorization for medical marijuana, it is pertinent to share basic facts of this anxiety disorder and the ways in which cannabis, as well as other treatments, can be helpful in the management of this condition.

A Patient Primer

A recent book by Bessel Van Der Kolk, M.D., titled *The Body Knows the Score—Brain, Mind, and Body in the Healing of Trauma* is the best review of our current understanding, or lack thereof, regarding how to help people heal from traumas. I recommend it particularly for patients who have been diagnosed with PTSD and for family members of those who suffer from PTSD.

As a specialist in pain management and addiction medicine with a longstanding interest in brain physiology, I shall share my perspective on trauma and healing. In my clinical work it is often quite pertinent.

In brief, PTSD shares a lot in common with all neurotic patterns, which we as humans are inclined to develop. As intelligent creatures we are very good at learning and not forgetting. We are understandably very good at remembering contexts in which life-threatening or traumatizing events have occurred. Without such abilities our survival as a species would be compromised. Most of our remembering is on a subconscious level, stemming in large part from less evolved areas of the primate brain. These less evolved areas are nonetheless essential because they play a primary role in ensuring survival and reproduction. If basic needs are threatened, our brains are designed to help us remember and learn from the experience. We learn what works and what does not.

By neurotic patterns I mean the apparent inability to forget old patterns of learning and response which are no longer useful. That is, as humans we continue to respond to cues or triggers which in the past have helped us to avoid harm, maintain the ability to reproduce, whether directly or indirectly, and to simply maintain our physiological homeostasis required for ongoing survival.

We all respond in the same way as the patient with PTSD. We expect the future to be similar to the past. If we are to be safe, we need to respond in customary ways. Indeed, if we deny the past or lessons learned, the consequences are apparent, and they play out on the world stage as well as in our individual lives. But the converse is true as well. If we are not able to adapt to new situations and we "neurotically" bring our old experiences and responses into the current ones, this too can be counterproductive and can warrant a label of illness as it does with PTSD.

The above perspective sees PTSD patterns as a spectrum of normal human response to memories of trauma. Similar to hypertension where blood pressure elevations are normal in response to a host of situational variables, it is the sustained and highly elevated responses that warrant our clinical attention. As with hypertension, the actual physiological findings of PTSD are not pathological and rarely produce immediate symptoms. Rather, the established neurotic patterns set the stage for or aggravate other conditions: cardiovascular problems, kidney problems, and visual problems. These are some of the best known long-term effects of hypertension. With PTSD we commonly see comorbid, anxiety-related issues such as insomnia and exaggerated startle responses. PTSD clearly contributes to pain levels as well as to responses to addictive substances. It is not coincidental that, as a pain management and addiction medicine specialist, I have developed skills in recognizing and treating PTSD patterns and patients.

For the sake of this discussion, I'm not limiting PTSD to patients who meet formal DSM 5 criteria for PTSD. As already mentioned, the patients who meet the formal criteria are likely at the more severe end of the spectrum to warrant immediate and effective care. In contrast to elevations in blood pressure, which are readily measured and objectified, the cut-off between acceptable levels and "pathological" levels of PTSD patterns are problematic and controversial.

Treatment Issues

For pragmatic reasons, as a physician I define treatable PTSD patterns as ones which are likely to contribute to other health and behavioral problems. What are the best treatments? Which are safest and most effective? As is the case with most conditions where objective biomarkers are lacking, the research to guide us is often lacking and professional opinions can vary significantly. Indeed, similar problems arise in all areas of mental illness where biomarkers are commonly lacking.

In terms of recommending treatments, I start with safety, accessibility, and the likelihood of benefits based on current understandings of brain function, research, and clinical experience. It is almost always best to individualize the elements of therapeutic planning; however, for educational purposes I shall share my current understanding on how to help brains function better. Indeed, in a recent article on "Mental Illness & Violence," I write of the pragmatic value of helping brains function better as a way of helping all forms of mental illness. I state:

"As to facts, it appears evident that brain function is what primarily directs complex human behavior. When behavior is not "healthy" the brain does not work well, whether because of inherent dysfunction or because of "contextual" variables such as lack of blood, nutrition, noise, toxins, etc. Of course, conditioning, and past events play an important role as well. The human brain is well designed to learn and remember.

The brain can be compared to a computer. Hardware and software contribute to the operation of both. However, unique hardware and software problems exist to make the brain quite different from a computer. In the brain hardware problems influence the software and can even change the software, and vice versa. Like a computer, if the input is defective, the output is also likely to be problematic. Because brains are made up of living cells, other factors can dramatically influence brain function. This leaves room for notions of the collective unconsciousness, spiritual factors, electrical fields, and just a whole lot of unknowns including the effects of love."

Treatment to be Medical, Behavioral, or Both?

Based on my above discussion about how brains operate, it is obvious that both medical and behavioral approaches will be commonly recommended. In the case of PTSD, both hardware and software components are likely to benefit from attention. Whether a given patient will respond optimally to one, or the other, or both is challenging to predict. As a result, I inevitably recommend a both/and approach.

Both non-specific and specific approaches exist in the medical as well as in the behavioral realms. By non-specific I mean those interventions which basically address the aroused fight-or-flight response often activated in patients with PTSD. In the medical arena, we utilize medicines that block sympathetic outflow, which can be blood pressure medicines and/or tranquilizers such as benzodiazepines or antidepressants. In the behavioral arena, we employ meditation techniques, yoga, spiritual practices, or cognitive behavioral therapy, demonstrated to be generally effective in reducing the fight-or-flight response. Some medicines, alternative therapeutic modalities, and behavioral approaches are deemed more likely be safe and effective to help in the context of PTSD. These are the ones commonly used. Behavioral approaches have been codified and widely available even in government publications looking at effective ways to address PTSD. I refer the reader to one linked on my website, "Dealing with the Effects of Trauma: A Self-Help Guide."

PTSD is categorized as an anxiety disorder. All medical and behavioral approaches which effectively address anxiety are likely to mitigate some of the signs and symptoms of PTSD. I have written recently on the subject of anxiety as a label in medicine and, while the discussion is somewhat academic, it might help one better appreciate the nature of PTSD and how we as a culture address it. "Anxiety—Just another Label?"

At this time, I consider cannabis and ketamine to be the most effective and therapeutic substances for PTSD. Both these agents inhibit activity in neural circuits involved in old traumatic memories. Ketamine at high dose is so effective in this regard that it is used as a dissociative agent in operating rooms. Glutamate (a neurotransmitter) levels also tend to be higher in some patients who are chronically stressed and agents that lower glutamate levels are another means to help some patients with PTSD.

One specific and well studied behavioral response to traumas that I am aware of is "Eye Movement Desensitization and Reprocessing (EMDR)." A skilled therapist can help the brain forget old patterns by initiating new cognitive images and meaning, which can be associated with traumatic memories and their associated current triggers or cues.

I am confident that other effective ways exist to address and help unlearn old neurotic patterns associated with past traumas. I know that certain specialists in acupuncture draw on techniques which can make dramatic differences. I am confident that other substances in addition to cannabinoids and ketamine could help. It is unlikely that formal research on the risks and benefits for cannabis or ketamine will happen soon because of the lack of financial incentives.

Life changing experiences have the potential to reset conditioned neural pathways. Occasionally, psychedelics have been used to elicit such responses. Ongoing spiritual pursuits, religious practices, and experiences of deep love can help reset longstanding neural pathways. One might include these experiences in potential non-specific interventions; however, I think it is better for them to be in their own class. With these experiences, something more transformative is going on than simply reducing anxiety or lowering the volume on the fight-or flight-response. It is as though the entire response pattern to past, real, or imagined threats has been altered, seemingly irrevocably. The individual can remain aware and benefit from past experiences, but the old patterns of response are changed in a substantive and generalized fashion.

Further discussion and links regarding PTSD can be found at DrRotchford.com under the "Handouts" tab.

CHAPTER FOUR

Preparing Cannabis for Medical Use

Cannabis for Oral (or Topical) Use

Rational medical use of cannabinoids warrants a mode of intake that is consistent with promoting both safety and effectiveness. Oral use (by mouth) or topically applied cannabinoids are arguably the best options regarding safety and effectiveness for medicinal purposes. An exception might be the patient receiving a chemotherapeutic agent who is expected to be nauseated or vomit shortly after dosing. As a result, high levels of cannabinoids which act quickly are indicated. In this context, smoking or "vaporizing" marijuana would be the best choice.

Advantages of Taking Cannabis by Mouth

- Longer duration of action

- Potentially more accurate and stable dosing

- Less likely to cause or aggravate addictive disorders

- Less likely to cause "spaciness" or sense of being "high." That is, a predominance of therapeutic actions rather than a "euphoric" or recreational effect. Also, probably less likely to cause other side effects such as paranoia.

- Avoids odors and other socially unacceptable effects of smoking.

• Avoids danger and risks to lungs of inhaling smoke and other risks associated with using "joints." (e.g. paper bi-products, glue bi-products, flaming oneself or other articles, stains, etc.)

Advantages of Smoking Cannabis

• More rapid onset of effect. If nauseated it avoids oral ingestion and has a faster result.

• Easier to dose to effect.

• Less expensive.

Given that medical marijuana is generally used for chronic conditions, smoking it for medicinal reasons in relatively contraindicated.

An online source for "edible" cannabis. Discussion is through Cannabis MD. Marijuana in Capsule Form, medmj-wa.com/ns-2.html

Using Glycerine to Prepare Cannabis for Oral Use

To be absorbed orally, that is by mouth, the active ingredients in marijuana (cannabinoids) need mixing with fats to allow better absorption into one's bloodstream. Historically, that is why one would put marijuana in brownies or butter. It is also why commercial oral forms generally involve gel caps with oils inside. The following is a method likely to be effective and allow for better, consistent dosing.

1. Purchase some *food quality* glycerine. Gallon containers are now online through Amazon.com and sell for around $25.00.

2. Depending upon the "potency" of the marijuana and how it is provided, crumble and pound leaves and buds into as fine a mixture as

possible. You may try using a coffee grinder. Sieve out bits of fiber and woody stalks. In Washington State in 2016 one can obtain "Baking Trim" marijuana for less than $4 per gram.

3. Using 14 grams of the sieved marijuana, put this in a quart cooking jar and add 500cc of the food quality glycerine.

4. Daily or twice daily, turn the bottle over to promote the cannabinoids being leached out into the glycerine fluid. Glycerine behaves like thick maple sugar and the cannabis tends to float to the top.

5. After a couple of weeks or so, the glycerine which was totally clear has turned a darker golden color. One may then strain the marijuana from the marijuana laced glycerine and keep this liquid in the refrigerator for stability. Warming the liquid can quicken the process, but heat also breaks down the cannabinoids and can increase the amount of psychoactive compounds.

6. The amount and potency of the marijuana used influences the potency of the liquid. If one uses marijuana with a THC potency of 15%, let us assume that 10% or more of the THC has leached into the glycerine. Since 10% of 14 grams is 1400 mg of THC, let us round things off to 1500 mg of THC as being assumed present for use in marijuana purported to have 15% THC concentrations.

7. If 1500mg are in 500cc of glycerine, this would mean that concentration is 3mg/ml of the final product. Using commercial grade Marinol as a comparison, most patients will respond best to divided doses in the range of 5mg to 30 mg per day.

8. Using the above estimates for concentration and dosing, one might start with one cc of the solution three times a day and work up gradually to a maximum of 3cc three times a day. Of course, if one "feels" something at the current dose, we would recommend lowering the dose similar to what we would do with a blood pressure medication.

9. One can find a one cc dispenser at any pharmacy. Using the above calculation and using 3cc to 9cc per day, the monthly cost including the cost of the 99.7% pure glycerine would be less than $10-30/month.

10. Note: Even in the best of laboratories struggle to determine accurately the concentration of THC or other cannabinoids. It has to do with cannabinoids being highly lipid soluble. In laboratory jargon this translates into the coefficient of variation between different measurements as being high. The implication is that all the above estimates for concentrations are rough estimates. Please assure clinical effectiveness through gradual dose adjustments. Avoid side-effects by assuring that levels are kept steady where one doesn't feel high or loaded, but rather one feels normal. It is the same as with taking a blood pressure medicine or an antidepressant. One can measure effects, and over time one might feel better and function better, but no feeling of a medication effect is associated directly with taking the medicine.

The above recipe has not been scientifically validated. Nonetheless, it provides effective clinical results, and it makes sense pharmacologically.

Rapid Extraction Method with Dry Ice

The following is a more rapid method for extracting hash (purified active ingredients) from the marijuana plant. Once the hash has been obtained, one could then dissolve the hash in any fat soluble liquid to obtain a stable dosing liquid to use. **Note: Cannabis in liquid form can also be used topically and can be very effective for some localized pain problems.**

More discussion, including YouTube shows about this method can be found online by doing a search for dry ice and cannabis. The following was extracted from one such online source.

"Not a particularly well-known method of making hash, dry ice hash has proven to be superior in both quantity as well as quality. It is extremely cost-effective and is perfect for growers who want to put their trimmings to use. You will need a bubble bag, a can or other container with diameter just smaller than the bubble bag's opening (a coffee can work about right), dry ice, large flat mirror or glass pane a hash press (not mandatory) and at least 1 ounce of trimmings.

First, place a piece of dry ice (about the size of a computer mouse) in the can or container. Place your trimmings and/or buds in the can on top of the piece of dry ice. Next, place a second piece of dry ice (about the same size) on top of the trimmings.

Next, secure the opening of the bubble bag over the opening of the can and make sure it fits tight and secure. You will want to get the can as far into the bag as possible.

Turn the can upside down so that the filtered screen on the bubble bag is over the center of your large glass pane. Begin to shake the can/bag directly over the glass. After about 30 seconds of shaking, you will notice a layer of kief begin to accumulate on the glass.

Keep shaking for 5 minutes. After this, stop shaking and remove any remaining chunks of dry ice from the can. Scrape the kief into a pile and place in your hash press.

A hash press can be purchased at any head shop (just be sure to ask for a pollen press). When pressed, this kief will become hash. You can also press it using paper by folding it and using your hands and body weight to firmly press the kief into hash. To get a lesser grade of hash, repeat the process with the trimmings you used the first time. You won't be disappointed with the amount of hash you can get out of these buds."

The THC4MS Recipe—Cannabis Chocolate

View recipe at THC4ms.org

Ingredients

150 grams dark chocolate (highest cocoa fat content possible)
3.5 grams of herbal cannabis

Utensils

1 pan
1 Pyrex bowl 1x
1 mold (ice-cube tray)
1 coffee grinder
1 sieve
1 plastic serving spoon

Method

Break chocolate up into small pieces and place in Pyrex bowl. Fill 1/3 of pan with water and bring to boil and then allow to simmer. Place Pyrex bowl in pan and allow chocolate to melt slowly, once melted continue to stir slowly.

Grind DRY herbal cannabis into a fine powder. Sieve out the bits of fiber and woody stalks. Grind again and sieve remains into the melted chocolate slowly, while stirring. DO NOT ALLOW PAN OF WATER TO BOIL DRY! Keep the bowl and mixture in the pan of water for at least 15 minutes, stirring occasionally over low heat.

Spoon the mixture into a suitable mold (ice cube tray works well) and allow to cool at room temperature before placing into the refrigerator for at least 6 hours. Remove chocolate by sharply banging the mold on a hard surface.

Some bars may have grayish edges due to fats from the chocolate separating out. This may be prevented by tempering (preheating and cooling) the chocolate.

CHAPTER FIVE

A QUITTER'S GUIDE

How to Recover from Marijuana and Other Addictions

We have already discussed various, potential side-effects of using medical cannabis and ways to mitigate these risks. Nevertheless, one side-effect occurring in 10-15% of patients who use cannabis regularly is the presence of a cannabis use disorder. As with opioid use disorders, the percentage of patients developing a substance use disorder is likely similar whether one uses cannabis for recreational or medicinal purposes. Both patients who are in the process of considering medical use of cannabis or who currently use cannabis for recreation will want to consider the potential for having or developing a substance use disorder and how to effectively recover from it.

Welcome To the Quitter's Guide

This workbook will help those who want to effectively address any addiction. While the workbook was initially designed with a focus on marijuana addiction, it is a valuable behavioral guide for addressing other addictions as well.

In conjunction with this workbook, we recommend the OPAS online handout "What Promotes Recovery from Addiction." While issues specific to treating marijuana addiction exist, we do emphasize general principles for treating addiction. We advise readers to use this workbook with a friend, sponsor, counselor, or loved one. We strongly advise against the tendency to remain in one's own head, or thinking that fending on one's own, is the best way.

The following is a brief list of elements associated with marijuana addiction not necessarily associated with other chemical addictions, possibly leading to some confusion.

• Persons envisioning recovery from marijuana addiction may need to battle the shame and consequences of having used what is still, based on federal law, an illicit substance.

• A false but common belief is that marijuana is not addictive.

• One may assume that its use is not to satisfy an addiction, but rather the use reflects medically approved or therapeutic purposes.

• Since the toxic effects of marijuana are significantly less than alcohol and are arguably less than tobacco, how could marijuana be that addictive?

• The serious consequences of marijuana use are not simply related to being "high" or under the influence. The consequences often relate to delayed and subtle effects. In contrast, people who drink alcohol are more likely to recognize direct and obvious consequences from inebriation: DUI's, poor choices, hangovers, to name a few.

- Similar to other therapeutic agents, marijuana when properly dosed and administered may help some brains function better. One might then mistakenly think, "Something that is helping my brain work better cannot be dangerous or addictive." Yet even pharmaceuticals, designed to treat specific brain diseases, can have serious and sometimes life-threatening side effects.

Indeed, marijuana is less addicting than most other abused substances. <u>Cannabis products</u> clearly produce less organ toxicity than alcohol or tobacco. Nonetheless, the consequences of marijuana addiction can be significant and, as the above list reflects, the challenges associated with accepting the diagnosis, are noteworthy.

Recovering from marijuana addiction is expected to be a life-long process as is true of other addictions. We recommend one take it one "step" and twenty-four hours at a time. The results will be self-evident!

We more easily accept change if the process feels positive. Recovery is not always fun, and by its nature patients can be expected to have uncomfortable feelings if not outright significant withdrawal symptoms. Overall, though, recovery is a decidedly positive undertaking. One can enjoy recovery. This workbook will support patients in that effort. It focuses on much more than just staying away from marijuana or other abused substances. It is also about doing new things and finding new rewards. If recovery is an ongoing struggle, we suggest you make changes to your plan.

Lastly, for any serious undertaking it is always helpful to have a formal plan. The best plans are tailored to the individual. Indeed, the best medical prescriptions are often individualized.

These plans have general goals, but they must also focus on specific actions necessary to help reach one's goals. For example, "Go to self-help groups" is a general goal. A specific action to reach that goal might be, "Go to a Narcotics Anonymous (NA) meeting Thursday evenings at seven and Saturday mornings at ten."

As we change how we respond to feelings, people, places, and things recovery becomes much more than "quitting." With the changes in behavior, the "stinking thinking" that often comes with drug use will begin to fade. At first, it is often helpful to "fake it until you make it." In other words, one does not have to understand the whys in order to experience the benefits of behavioral changes. One can act in new ways because that is what one was advised to do. Eventually, however, one begins to understand and reap the benefits. One's view of recovery and of the world will change. All aspects of one's life will improve. This is the hidden blessing of all successful recoveries.

Most recovering people have heard the saying,"If you do what you have always done, you will get what you have always gotten." But it works the other way, too. If one changes what one does, and it is for the better, progress and better experiences inevitably follow. The slogan "Fake it until you make it" is not so much to be understood as practiced, and then experienced.

This workbook includes recommended assignments. These assignments are not prescriptions! In recovery, it is best to remember: "Take what's of use and leave the rest!" All the best to you and yours.

Look at How Use Affects Your Life—Get Motivated!

While inevitably better in the long run to keep your sights on what one wants to see happen, early on it can be helpful to review some of the downsides of using marijuana.

Marijuana and substance abuse may alter your perceptions, judgment and reasoning ability. It is therefore difficult for one to know whether the substance is affecting performance in work or school. For example, it is not uncommon for marijuana users to assume that the drug even helps them excel at certain tasks for that is how it "feels." But one must seriously ask oneself, "Am I having problems in relationships, or social, legal, school or work concerns? How am I doing financially?" If one's brain is functioning as well as it can, most likely one can hope to see progress in all dimensions of one's life. With some reflection, this makes common sense.

The first assignment is to enhance motivation for change. When we focus on core values and base our behavior accordingly, the motivation which follows is often the strongest and most enduring.

Assignment 1—Questions to review one's use and values.

Many people have never formerly examined, or expressed, their fundamental values. It is essential to recognize what one truly values! Come up with at least three basic values before answering the following questions. It helps to ask others what their most cherished values are. By so doing, our own values may become clearer. Values can and do change. It is helpful to know what they are currently so as to best leverage them in your present stage of recovery.

Check either yes or no.

1. In general do you see marijuana/substance use helping you live your life consistent with your values?   Yes ____   No ____

2. Do you relate better to people who smoke marijuana or abuse substances than to people who do not abuse substances, and if so, is this consistent with your values?   Yes ____   No ____

3. Do you find yourself thinking about marijuana or other substances more often than you would like?   Yes ____   No ____

4. Have you stopped doing healthy things because of marijuana/substance use? (e.g. exercising, eating, sleeping, working, or following advice from those committed to your health)

          Yes ____   No ____

5. Have you avoided medical recommendations because of marijuana or substance use?   Yes ____   No ____

6. Have you ever noticed while smoking marijuana that you cannot remember what you just read or were told?

          Yes ____   No ____

7. Have you spent much time thinking about how you could make money by growing, distributing, or selling marijuana?

          Yes ____   No ____

9. Do you find that you ever "sneak" or are dishonest about marijuana use? Yes ___   No ___

10. Have concerns arisen about causing undue worry or harm to those you care about as the result of use? Yes ___   No ___

11. Do you prefer the feeling of being stoned over most other ways of feeling? Yes ___   No ___

12. Does the use of marijuana or other substances affect your choices about work or entertainment? Yes ___   No ___

13. Are you having social, financial, or legal problems because of marijuana/substance use ? Yes ___   No ___

14. Have you checked your hepatitis C status knowing that marijuana use is more dangerous if you have this disease?

Yes ___   No ___

15. Have you or other people expressed concerns about your friends, that your motivation has decreased, or that you've become less productive in your endeavors? Yes ___   No ___

16. Have you felt anxious, irritable, or had headaches or difficulty sleeping when you went several days without smoking marijuana or using a substance? Yes ___   No ___

17. Has there been someone in your life who you have loved, or who you have truly liked, who you do not see anymore because of your marijuana use? Yes ___   No ___

Yes responses indicate that marijuana use may be part of a problem rather than a solution and most importantly may not be consistent with your values. Review with someone trustworthy, who is not invested in whether you smoke or not, about looking at your relationship with marijuana and its possible consequences. If everything is getting better in your life, your health, your relationships, your finances, legal concerns, etc.; it is likely that marijuana is not a serious concern. Some yes answers to the above do, however, warrant attention.

Assignment 2—Substance use may interfere with reaching goals

Has marijuana/substance use kept you from getting anything you wanted in life? Did the use of marijuana interfere with your reaching a goal? Write three examples here.

1.

2.

3.

Make a Plan for Recovery—Make it your own!

Planning ahead as we already emphasized is essential for a successful recovery. That means choosing—in advance—how and when you will respond to people, places, and things. Without a plan, it is most likely that a slip or relapse will occur. Someone who does not plan is trying to use the old willpower model to stay clean. The reasoning goes something like this: if I'm tough enough and strong enough, I can just tough it out through recovery. I do not have to change anything else about my life—I just will not use marijuana. Or, I will not use it for a while. Or, I'll use it less than I used to.

Hopefully, one is able to accept that with addictions willpower does not cut it. What's needed is an active strategy for recovery. If one wants to succeed in recovery, make a plan. Then put the same amount of effort into the plan as one did into using. Twelve-step programs lay out a tried and true plan, one step at a time. While it is a powerful and effective program, 12-step programs do not work for everyone. Find out what works. Learning from the experience of others is always a healthy bet!

Be Prepared to Problem-Solve

How does one go about solving problems related to relationships, feelings, people, places, and things? Often it depends on the context. Here are principles or steps found to be of help to others.

1. Define the problem.

2. Think of possible solutions.

3. Pragmatic or workable solutions are often the best.

4. Write a list of "to dos" to accomplish that solution, and schedule a time for each item on the list.

5. Practice the solutions in your mind.

6. Benefit from outside input.

An example will be demonstrative: one is planning to attend a funeral. Already feelings of anxiety start to come up. One expects further uncomfortable feelings to come up during the funeral. Friends and family members who still use will likely be there. Furthermore, a wake has been planned for after the funeral. More than likely, opportunities will arise to go outside and share a joint. This is a clear set up for a slip. It is a time to have a plan. It is time to grab a pencil and paper to make some notes.

Then go through the six problem-solving steps.

1. Define the problem.

In this case, the problem is a friend will likely want to share a joint. It will be difficult to say no.

2. Think of possible solutions.

a. Choose not to attend the funeral or the wake.

b. Attend the funeral and not go to the wake.

c. Invite a clean and sober friend. Just by being there, the friend would strengthen the choice not to use. Let other friends or family members know of the plans not to use. Even ask for suggestions!

3. Choose the most workable solution. Solution c sounds best. It allows attendance at the funeral and wake. At the same time, it increases the chances of staying clean & sober. Furthermore, learning how to grieve and not use is a vital skill to learn. To process grief with others is most always a healthy plan.

4. Write a list of "to do's" to accomplish that solution and schedule a time for each item on the list. As an example:

• Plan two phone calls, one to a friend and another to any understanding soul who will be attending. Be as specific as possible about the timing of the calls.

•

•

•

5. Rehearse the solution

During the days before the funeral, pretend one is a theatrical director and lay out how one will "act" at the funeral and reception. Know what lines might be helpful to use. To visualize the events is all the better! It is as if the event will be a pleasant and successful dream. See oneself at the reception with the supportive friend. See oneself laughing, eating, and enjoying being with people. When an old smoking buddy strikes up a conversation, introduce your clean and sober friend. Seek out relatives or friends who are less likely to trigger cravings. A plan to "reward" oneself after the reception for remaining clean and sober can be helpful. Perhaps a movie, a special meal, or time with a friend, could act as powerful and sustaining rewards?

6. Share your plan with another. Get some input. Take what's of use and leave the rest. Do not assume one is supposed to have all the answers and be prepared for the anxiety that is likely to come up. Whoever one talks with will preferably validate your feelings as being entirely normal. The lesson here is that, while uncomfortable feelings come up, this is not an excuse to use! It is an opportunity to learn new ways to respond to uncomfortable feelings.

Keep these six steps in mind for all sorts of problem solving. Any successful business uses similar ones. The assignments below will help one implement the steps and chart a positive recovery course. One begins to respond in constructive ways to the people, places, and things in one's life—instead of letting them or one's feelings control one's behavior. These skills will help one to be successful in all sorts of endeavors.

Assure adequate medical care or screening

Access to specialized care in addiction medicine is sorely lacking. Some medications can help in early recovery to marijuana and other substance addictions. With some addictions, medications can be essential and lifesaving. This is particularly the case with opiates, but also with alcohol and other sedatives. Many medical and psychiatric conditions may interfere with a recovery. Chronic painful conditions are a common complicating medical condition. Mood disorders, anxiety disorders, PTSD, ADHD are common psychiatric conditions. Other addictions are also often involved. Addictions associated with licit substances such as alcohol or tobacco and even prescription medications are quite common. Addictions to illicit substances are also common. It is also easy to overlook "relationship addictions" or other behavioral addictions. Current relationships and attachments to them are possibly the biggest impediment to a successful recovery. The term "relationship addict" has even been coined, and further information is available online and in print.

Ask your physician for a medical and psychiatric evaluation in view of your addiction to marijuana or other substances. If they appear uneasy or they have no helpful suggestions, ask for a suitable referral.

Use your new problem solving skills to assure that treatable medical and psychiatric conditions are not interfering with recovery.

Avoidance Is Sometimes Helpful

Avoidance is clearly a reasonable solution early on in recovery. Why make it more difficult than it need be? A failure to change the people, places, and things that promote drug use is often a clear set up for a relapse. While avoidance is not the best long-term plan, early in recovery triggers for relapse are powerful. Always assume that subconscious triggers that prompt use are prevalent. These triggers are present even years after one is clean and sober. We can now observe in the brains of people who have been clean and sober for years, dramatic changes that occur when confronted with known triggers. These changes in brain activity occur without any conscious awareness of them! Recognizing and having plans for known triggers is the heart of relapse prevention. It's the "what do I do when my friend offers me a toke as we are walking into a dance?"

Even after years of successful recovery when people feel reassured they will never again use, these subconscious drives are cunning, baffling, and powerful. The good news is they do lose their power. After having successfully navigated through the situations which formerly would trigger use or bring up cravings, one can attend a wedding, funeral, or even have a visit from a using friend and be surprised by how easy and even enjoyable it can be. Feelings of gratitude can emerge that fill one up as well as friends and family. This is just one of the payoffs of recovery.

It is best, though, to assume the subconscious cues continue to lurk in the subconscious. Typical examples are grief or resentments not thoroughly recognized or processed. Reasons exist for the slogan "One day at a time."

Shame about feeling ashamed about one's lack of control will slowly vanish. In 12-step programs this is in part what the first step is trying to promote. The first step which addresses one's lack of control benefits from regular reminders. One easy way to explain why one cannot be around certain people, places, or things is to openly acknowledge, "I can't handle it at this time, and I'm working at it!" Paradoxically, these can be very empowering statements.

Assignment 3—Emulate sober and clean people you respect.

Find one or two clean and sober people whom you respect and admire. Try to be like them. If one intends to emulate someone, it helps to spend some time with them. In doing this, one has the possibility to better know what makes them tick.

Who are some of these people you would like to spend time with? **Make a list.**

-

-

-

Use the above problem solving skills to figure out how and when to contact them. Once contacted, schedule some time with them ASAP.

Assignment 4—Consider Professional Counseling

Professional counseling is helpful for many. Since marijuana or other substance use can subtly affect the way one thinks and responds to feelings, professional counselors can point out some of the learned patterns and suggest others. Getting professional counseling can also help one to see the "Big Picture" about using. We routinely recommend professional counseling for the benefits likely outweigh the risks and cost.

List at least three people who might be called/asked.

1.

2.

3.

If you don't know of any counseling resources, then list the names of three people who could help you think of some options.

1.

2.

3.

How and when will you contact a potential counselor?

Do you need help to arrange counseling? Often one needs to figure out how to afford, how to get transportation, and confront other barriers. If so, list the name of someone who could provide some input regarding these barriers to further care.

•

When and how will you contact this person?

•

Anxiety often accompanies the idea of seeing a counselor. The first visit has three primary questions to answer: Do you feel safe with this person? Did you feel respected and validated? Do they get it?

Assignment 5—Find new places to hang out.

Most substance abusers use in private as well as public places. You might have used at home in the morning or evening, or perhaps in your car. Or you might have used in a parking lot at work or school. List the places where you most often smoked marijuana or abused your substance.

•

•

•

•

Underline the places you can avoid during your early recovery. These are to be expected to be triggers for relapse. Circle the places you cannot avoid.

Now imagine yourself with a chance to use in one of the places you circled. What can you say or do to avoid using? List each place you circled; then write down some phrases you could say or actions you could take.

-

-

-

Have alternatives for what you intend to do in these places instead of using? List at least three options here.

1.

2.

3.

Assignment 6—Find a self-help group

How or why self-help groups work are questions frequently asked by someone contemplating going. Even without a satisfactory response, be sure to at least to give it a college try. After the 2nd or 3rd time attending a group, one often feels better than one felt before. That confirms it might be helping for reasons yet to be appreciated.

Are you attending any self-help groups, such as NA, AA or Alanon? List those groups here.

-
-

If you are not attending any self-help groups, then do you know of any in your area? List them here.

-
-

Do you know where and when these groups meet? If so, list the times and locations for each group. (If you don't know of meetings, check the phone book.) Then, list a contact person for each group. Write each person's name and phone number next to his or her group listing.

If you do not know of any groups in your area, then who can help you find that information? List some names here or check it out through the internet.

-
-
-
-

Choose one name to begin with and then figure out how and when you will contact this group..

Assignment 7—Fun and social activities are important

List some recreational activities that do not involve addictive substances. Activities which involve others are often the best. Consider playing or learning a sport. If one plays an instrument, find someone to play along with. If one sings, consider joining a choir. Perhaps learning something new and fun sounds appealing. Volunteer and service work helps those doing it perhaps more than those they serve. Take advantage of a faith tradition when present.

List a couple activities here.

-

-

-

Look at the list. Circle any activities you would enjoy doing now.

Now choose one of the activities you circled. If you wanted to do this activity, what steps would you need to take? List the activity and the steps you would take. Whom would you need to contact? What equipment or materials would you need?

-

-

Which of the above steps can you complete in the coming week? List them here, along with a specific time for doing each of them.

-

-

-

Assignment 8—Your brain requires good nutrition and exercise

In large part, recovery is about getting the old brain working right. Proper food and exercise really help.

Making a recovery plan gives one the chance to look at how and what you eat. This is an excellent time to make changes in one's diet which promote overall health. Eating habits, changes in moods, can all be triggers for substance use. When one makes a positive change in one of these areas, it can affect other positive changes.

The brain likes structure and regularity. Consider scheduling regular meals, sleep, and wake-up times.

Make a list of one or two changes one intends to make in the way one eats or drinks (for example, switching to low-fat foods, drinking decaffeinated coffee, or more fruit and vegetables). Remember to keep it simple.

When one craves snacks, find a substitute for eating. For example, instead of eating a dessert or drinking a cup of coffee after dinner, consider listening to some music, going for a walk, or calling a friend.

List one or two activities, which could work for you.

-

-

Do you exercise regularly? If so, describe your exercise routine here.

-

If you aren't exercising regularly, then list some possible forms of exercise you could start within the next week. Remember the slogans "easy does it," "it takes time," "progress not perfection." These slogans are all helpful reminders, when initiating a new exercise program.

Now choose one type of exercise that would be fun or at least possibly fun for you. List it here.

-

What steps can you take to begin this activity? For example, do you need equipment, supplies, training? How will you get those things? What exactly will you do? When? Where? With whom?

At DrRotchford.com under the handouts tab, you can also find a handout entitled "Brain Health 101," which contains further clues to help your brain work better.

Assignment 9—Plans for staying sober at school or work

School or work-related settings can be triggers.

Are you aware of any which could be triggers? When you work too hard, do you feel like you deserve some "time off?" What school or work activities tend to justify use?

List the triggers you are aware of related to work or school.

-

-

What are your options/plans for responding differently? Remember to use your new problem-solving skills.

-

-

Do you have access to an employee assistance program or a student assistance program? If so, you are fortunate. Consider making an appointment with that counselor this week. Put your plan in writing here.

-

Assignment 10—Plans for staying sober with family

Another common setting for triggers are those associated with family events. A fight with a spouse, partner, children, or even a neighbor is likely to trigger cravings. Sometimes family reunions or holidays generate anxiety. One can use just to feel more comfortable at family reunions. It would be rare if one were not triggered by some family affair.

The plan is to have a strategy and to use one's problem solving skills. One can change the way one thinks or feels about family related triggers, and it takes time and persistence. Some suggestions include: take a course to sharpen your listening or communication skills, discuss family problems with a family counselor or a friend. Lastly, and perhaps most importantly, ask family members to become familiar with addiction issues and encourage them to attend ALANON or other self-help groups for family members.

List options for reducing family cues for relapse

-
-
-

From the actions listed, choose one that you can complete in the next month. Step by step, describe what you will do and when you will do it.

-
-
-
-

Assignment 11—Problem-solving regarding cravings

Many sights, sounds, smells, or thoughts trigger cravings for marijuana or other addictive substances. Even listening to music may trigger cravings and an urge to use. One cannot directly control the strength of any craving. One can, though, take some steps to change one's response to a craving. Develop a detailed picture in your mind about what to do when a craving comes up. Keep the following points in mind.

- It is normal to feel cravings.

- Cravings do not last. By nature, they will pass. Physiological correlates to cravings exist, and it is likely with time medications will arise which interfere with cravings. Until then, these behavioral suggestions are what we have to offer and most likely will always remain helpful.

- The craving feels most intense just before it starts to fade.

When one gives in to a craving and uses, the next craving could be stronger. If one does not give in to cravings to use, over time the cravings tend to become weaker

Again, do some problem solving around how to deal with cravings. For the next few days, pay attention to any cravings. Answer the following questions.

- When did you feel cravings? List specific times.

- Where were you when you felt cravings?

- What were you doing when you felt cravings?

- Now look at the big picture. Do you see patterns in your cravings? For example, do you feel more intense cravings on certain days or at certain times? Do certain people, places, or things seem associated with strong cravings? Describe any patterns you see.

-

-

-

Now decide how you want to respond to cravings. Here are some ideas that have worked for other people on the journey of recovery.

- Write a brief message to give yourself when you feel a craving.

- Attempt to identify the feeling that prompted the craving. HALT stands for Hungry, Angry, Lonely, and Tired. Once the feeling is acknowledged and respected, it often subsides. Talking with an understanding listener about how one is feeling can also make a big difference.

- Choose a prayer, slogan, or quotation you are fond of. Make sure it is positive and recovery-oriented. Memorize this message and recite it silently or aloud. Consider writing the message on a card and carry it with you.

- Take a specific action when you feel a craving. If certain music triggers cravings for you, then play different music. Choose an alternative action that is easy to do in a variety of times and places. For example, some people find it helpful to take long, slow, deep breaths when cravings occur.

• Recall to mind a specific time when you felt your recovery was going exceptionally well. Pretend you made a videotape of that situation. Now in your mind play back the videotape. Where were you, and who were you with? What were you doing? What were you saying? What thoughts were running through your mind? Recall as many details as you can. Make the picture in your mind as bright and colorful as possible.

• Often we will do for others what we might not do for ourselves. Carry with you a small picture of someone you love. Choose someone with a stake in your recovery—a spouse, partner, child, parent, or friend. Look at this picture whenever you feel cravings. This can remind you that staying clean and sober involve others as well as yourself.

Now think of some things you can do when you recognize a craving. List at least six possibilities here.

1.

2.

3.

4.

5.

6.

Choose an option to try for a week. Describe exactly what you will do.

Keep a Journal

When we write things down, we are more likely to pay attention. Most of us have fleeting thoughts that flood our waking hours. This makes it problematic to stay focused on any one thing. Writing it down helps us pay attention and to focus on solutions.

Often the best plans are written plans. After your plan is down on paper you can add to it, change it, and refine it. Keeping a journal is a popular practice among many recovering people. This activity gives you regular access to your important thoughts and feelings.

You don't have to write well to keep a journal. Nobody else needs to read it. Write every day, and remember no specific format is necessary to follow. Just do what works.

Here are some ways to get started with a journal.

- List your recovery "to dos." A typical entry might be "Three things I need to do to stay sober today." Before you go to sleep, review your list and jot down some thoughts for the next day.

- Keep lists—gratitude lists, inventories, or amends you have made or need to make.

- One month from now, go through these assignments again. Write your new responses in your journal. Doing so facilitates progress and refinement of your plan.

- Write out prayers, meditations, and slogans you like, or create your own.

- Sum up key insights about recovery that you've discovered from reading books, listening to tapes, or talking with other recovering

Start a journal now following one of the suggestions given.

Assignment 12—Review regularly what you have learned

Recovery is not a straight-line process and clearly involves more than abstinence. Recovery is circular or helix like in its progression. One advances while frequently returning to similar concerns or steps. One might be in a very successful recovery program and not be entirely abstinent. Patients who are on agonist therapy for opioid addiction are the classic example. It is most difficult to make significant progress while still self-medicating with a substance. Nonetheless, it is well understood that stages of change occur well before one actually stops using. So, one might be changing and not even recognize it!

After reviewing this workbook, list the three most important things you have learned about yourself.

1.

2.

3.

Now list the three most important actions you are willing to take as part of your recovery plan. These are actions you intend to carry out no matter what.

1.

2.

3.

Review this list from time to time to make sure your recovery plan is on track. Then savor all the positive changes that recovery is bringing to your life. As the old slogan reminds us, "Keep it simple." People falter in recovery when they make it too complicated. This workbook attempts to help break recovery down into simple principles and behavioral changes. Remember the "Fake it until you make it" slogan and know that it is based on solid understandings of how our brains best learn new patterns.

We are designed to remember and to remember well. Our actual survival often depends upon it. So rather than focus on "forgetting" our past behaviors, go with the flow and help your brain start to remember new and healthier ways of responding. With time the new ways will crowd out the old ways. I advise rather than trying to tune out an old dysfunctional radio program, it works best to focus on a really lively and rewarding movie. In view of keeping it simple, consider learning these five tips. One for each finger.

Tips To Help Maintain Your Recovery

Tip 1—Develop a clear picture of what you want to happen

Formulate as clear of a picture as you can of how your life will be as a result of a robust recovery. What will you do, say, and how might you think differently? How would you act and feel if you did not experience any toxic shame? What would it look like if uncomfortable feelings were addressed in ways that didn't involve substance use? If you've done the assignments in this workbook, you've already got lots of answers to these questions. You've started to bring the future you are looking for into a clearer focus.

Tip 2—Be willing to change

If the changes you are envisioning are consistent with your basic values, you are set. By definition, you are willing to change. Additionally, as the Big Book of AA points out, "What we need is the honesty, openness, and willingness to start changing. In time, the rest will follow."

Tip 3—We are affected by our environment and relations

Surround yourself by loving and caring people. Be around those who have successfully navigated recovery. Learn and benefit from their mistakes as well as their successes. Involve others in your recovery. There's no need to go it alone. Indeed, that is often a recipe for disaster.

Reach out and ask for support. It makes all the difference. Asking for help and persisting in asking is highly predictive for a successful recovery.

Tip 4—Keep at it

Many people make the mistake of thinking they have learned all they need to know. They mistakenly think it is all behind them and they are back in control. The nature of addiction is that over time and with the proper triggers, slips or relapses are waiting to happen. Keep at it. Keep learning about addiction and what works and what does not. There will be ups, there will be downs. Keep at it and serenity follows.

Tip 5—Do what it takes

Sometimes it is as simple as calling a sponsor and having him or her remind you, "Don't use, keep going to meetings, and this too shall pass." Sometimes it is a prayer, sometimes remembering the feelings of gratitude one has experienced. It is no wonder that 12-step programs include the phrase "These are but suggestions." Those savvy about addiction recognize that no one shoe will fit everyone. But do not be confused. This does not mean that sound and solid principles and steps do not exist. This workbook has the intent to convey helpful principles and steps to take.

Further References

In addition to the already noted references, numerous references are now available on the web. Dr. Rotchford has put together references related to addiction on his website at <u>DrRotchford.com</u>. Look under the "Handouts" tab for articles, which might be of interest.

GLOSSARY

Medical Cannabis—Definitions and Terminology

A comprehensive list is available at <u>ColoradoPotGuide.com</u>

Anandamide: one of the body's naturally occurring cannabinoids.

Bioavailability: a measure of the proportion of a drug that is absorbed. Most cannabinoids ingested by mouth have a bioavailability of 10 to 20 percent. Inhaled, they're 30 to 50 percent. Bioavailability of cannabinoids are highly influenced by the fat content of the food or vehicle it is consumed with. Cannabinoids are fat soluble.

Butane hash oil: very concentrated cannabinoid-rich oil that is made by using butane to extract cannabinoids from cannabis plants. CO_2 and other solvents can be used.

Cannabidiol (CBD): one of several dozen naturally occurring cannabinoids. It binds only weakly to CB1 and CB2 receptors in the brain and does not cause the "high" feelings associated with THC.

Cannabidiolic acid: the acidic form of CBD in plants before harvest—converted to active CBD by drying and heat. Cannabigerol

(CBG): a naturally occurring cannabinoid that is not psychoactive, but speculatively may slow abnormal cancer growth.

Cannabinoids: a group of molecules that exist in cannabis plants and can also be synthesized in a laboratory.

Cannabis: the genus of the marijuana-producing plant, which includes the species *Cannabis sativa* and *Cannabis indica*. Disagreement exists about whether a third group, *Cannabis ruderalis*, is a separate species. It appears that the overlap in genetic code between the different species is now immense because of cross fertilizing, etc. One strain of sativa may have more in common with an indica strain and vice versa. The difference in genetic code between different strains may be as great as those differences between apes and humans.

CB1 receptors: cannabinoid receptors on neurons in the brain and on cells in the male & female reproductive systems, and elsewhere.

CB2 receptors: cannabinoid receptors on microglial cells in the brain and on immune cells. High densities of these receptors occur where concentrations of white blood cells are found (e.g. in the spleen and gastrointestinal tract).

Concentrates: substances with very high levels of cannabinoids: oil, wax, shatter, butter, hash, and many others.

Dispensary: in Washington State the designation for a licensed business that sells marijuana products.

Dronabinol: a synthetic form of THC, given by mouth, available by prescription. It's trade name is Marinol. Though it is synthetic (manmade), one can assume that, because it's properties are identical to THC, it acts in similar ways. Because it is a pharmaceutical, it has the distinct advantage of being more reliable as to concentrations and doses.

Edibles: foods that have been infused with marijuana extracts and that contain THC, CBD, and other cannabinoids.

11-0H-tetrahydrocannabinol (11-0H-THC): a metabolite of THC, it is produced in the liver and is at least as psychoactive as THC. 11-nor-9-carboxy-THC is also a metabolite of THC, but is not psychoactive.

First-pass effect: the metabolic "tax" that the liver imposes on a drug taken by mouth, by altering the drug's structure, often making it inactive. (Drugs absorbed through the lining of the mouth or inhaled bypass the direct effect of the liver).

Green Dragon: high-proof alcohol that has been infused with marijuana.

Hash: a concentrated form of marijuana, consisting mostly of cannabinoid-rich trichomes from a cannabis plant.

Herbal marijuana: herbs that may have psychoactive properties, often laced with synthetic cannabinoids.

Indica: *Cannabis indica* is a separate species of cannabis that has different properties, but each source or strain is likely to be significantly different from another.

Marinol: see Dronabinol above.

Nabilone: a synthetic cannabinoid developed in the 1970s and still used for the treatment of nausea.

Permeation enhancers: chemicals like dimethylsulfoxide (DMSO) that help cannabinoid molecules pass through the skin or other barriers to fat soluble absorption.

Pistils: small, hair-like fibers found on female cannabis plants that have high cannabinoid concentrations.

Placebo marijuana: marijuana from which cannabinoids were removed—the way caffeine is removed from coffee beans.

Sativa: *Cannabis sativa* is a separate species of cannabis. While "pure" strains have properties different than "pure" strains of indica, the overlaps are significant.

Shatter: a form of marijuana concentrate that has the consistency of glass.

Stamen: part of a flower used to identify male buds; it is low in THC and CBD and thus often culled.

Synthetic cannabinoids: artificial molecules that share some properties with naturally occurring cannabinoids. Recently, they have been more commonly abused and are associated with unique side effects properties.

Tetrahydrocannabinol (THC): the most common cannabinoid in marijuana. It is responsible for marijuana's psychoactive effects. When carboxylated, primarily through heating, it produces the associated psychoactive effects of marijuana. Metabolites of THC also have some psychoactive properties, but generally raw, uncooked marijuana plants, juiced and consumed in quantity, have marginal if any psychoactive effects.

Tetrahydrocannabinolic acid: the acidic (and inactive) form of THC present in plants before they're harvested. It's converted to THC by drying and heat.

Tincture: cannabinoids dissolved in ethanol or fat soluble solutions such as glycerine or coconut-based oils. Tinctures are consumed by mouth.

2-Arachidonoylglycerol: an endocannabinoid, like anandamide, which binds to the body's cannabinoid receptors.

Vaporizer: a device used to convert to vapor the cannabinoids in marijuana in order to be inhaled. This mode of delivery reduces some of the irritant effects on the airways of smoking cannabis.

Wax: a highly concentrated form of cannabinoids that has a gooey consistency.

RESOURCES

Learn About Reform of Marijuana Law in Washington State

The University of Washington's Alcohol & Drug Abuse Institute provides current and science-based information about marijuana with a specific emphasis on knowledge focusing on the state of Washington.

Access factsheets and resources at adai.washington.edu/marijuana/.

Political Action

Attitudes and laws regarding the use of marijuana are political. If one is interested in ending the "War on Drugs" policies of our federal government, perhaps the most active and credulous national organization is the Drug Policy Alliance Network. They are at DrugPolicy.org/homepage.cfm

Additional Online information

The NIDA Facts

drugabuse.gov/publications/drugfacts/marijuana

A host of reputable and helpful information on marijuana is available on the internet. While the government has its own biases, for many reasons the National Institute on Drug Abuse (NIDA) site is more likely than most sites to contain "objective" facts regarding marijuana.

Partnership for Drug-Free Kids has a site regarding the latest news on addiction and policy, found at DrugFree.org/join-together. At no cost, they provide helpful subscriber email lists. As their name suggestions, they have implied biases. The evidence is overwhelming, however, that cannabis use in youth is particularly risky.

Cannabis Medical Dictionary

CannabisMD.squarespace.com

Cannabis Tolerance

With chronic cannabis use, tolerance develops to the physiological (i.e.cardiovascular) and subjective (i.e.highness) effects.

Benowitz NL, Jones RT J Clin Pharmacol. 1981 Aug-Sep; 21(8-9 Suppl):214S-223S.

Hart CL, Haney M, Ward AS, Fischman MW, Foltin RW Drug Alcohol Depend. 2002 Aug 1; 67(3):301-9.

Books

Baum, Dan, *Smoke and Mirrors: The War on Drugs and the Politics of Failure*, Little, Brown & Co, 1996

Cermak, Timmen, *Marihuana: What's a Parent to Believe?* Hazelden, 2003

Earlywine, Mitch, *Understanding Marihuana*, Oxford University Press, 2002

Video Programs

YouTUBE is a wonderful resource on which videos can be viewed. Do a search for "medical cannabis" to bring up videos produced by anyone from physicians to people who suffer from substance abuse. Many videos are educational. Some are of questionable value. Be discerning and make up your own mind as to what videos have value for your interests and needs. Dr. Rotchford produced a series of 12 YouTUBE videos on opioid use for patients. View videos on DrRotchford.com/videos

Other Resources

Recommended resources for further information on the topic of medical cannabis are TED Talks and Wikipedia. Do a search on each for "medical cannabis" for a list of topical subjects to pursue. Many online websites delve deeply into subjects related to medical cannabis. A good site at which to start is leafly.com.

About the Author

J. Kimber Rotchford, M.D., M.P.H., has longstanding expertise in treating patients who suffer from chronic pain, addictions, and related disorders. Dr. Rotchford is among the first pain management specialists certified by the American Academy of Integrative Pain Management. Since 1981, he has emphasized and implemented integrative approaches to pain management.

Passionate about finding effective and practical solutions for managing chronic pain, Dr. Rotchford became a specialist in medical acupuncture and addiction medicine. He is a Fellow of the American Academy of Medical Acupuncture and is one of the first physicians to be board certified in addiction medicine through the American Board of Addiction Medicine. The author of professional publications related to pain management and addiction medicine, he was among the first physicians to authorize marijuana for medical uses in Washington State, in 1998.

Dr. Rotchford has a strong background in public health and is a long-standing Fellow of the American College of Preventive Medicine. A native of Washington, he is a graduate of the University of Washington's School of Medicine and School of Public Health. The University of Washington has a noteworthy history of leadership and expertise in both chronic pain management and public health. He has also studied, worked, and taught internationally.

Recognized for his compassion and his expertise in the treatment of chronic pain and opioid use disorders, Dr. Rotchford has practiced exclusively in small towns in Washington State. First, he served patients along Washington's Pacific Coast. For the past 25 years, he has practiced medicine in Port Townsend, Washington. Dr. Rotchford's full curriculum vitae is online at DrRotchford.com/resume.

About the Editors

Dan Youra publishes and edits books and magazines on health topics. He is the editor of 420 Flagship.com, founded by Youra Tarverdi with Bloom Innovations, Nug, and Agre Holdings to promote the responsible sales of cannabis products in California's dispensaries.

Andie Mitchell is a freelance writer and editor. She also works in garden restoration and design. She lives in Port Townsend, WA with her family.

OTHER BOOKS BY THE AUTHOR

Opioids In Chronic Pain Management
A Guide For Patients

Opidemic – A Public Health Epidemic

Books for sale on Amazon and at retail stores.

Olympas Medical Services
J. Kimber Rotchford, M.D., M.P.H.

Olympas Pain and Addiction Services Clinic
1136 Water St. Suite 107
Port Townsend, WA 98368
www.OPAS.us
staff@OPAS.us

Made in the USA
Columbia, SC
07 June 2018